Chapter 1: Introduction to Aromatic Alchemy

The History of Essential Oils

The history of essential oils can be traced back thousands of years, with their use documented in ancient civilizations such as Egypt, China, and India. The Egyptians utilized these aromatic compounds not only for their delightful fragrances but also for their therapeutic and preservative properties. Essential oils were integral to their religious rituals, embalming processes, and skincare practices. The famous Ebers Papyrus, dating back to 1550 BC, reveals a wealth of knowledge about the use of aromatic plants for medicinal purposes, indicating the early recognition of the healing potential of essential oils.

In ancient China, essential oils were embraced in traditional medicine, where they were used to promote wellness and balance within the body. The practice of aromatherapy has roots in Chinese medicine, emphasizing the concept of Qi, or life force energy. Essential oils derived from plants were believed to enhance this energy, contributing to physical and emotional well-being. Meanwhile, in India, the practice of Ayurveda incorporated essential oils into its holistic approach, using them in various treatments to achieve harmony among body, mind, and spirit. These ancient practices laid the groundwork for the modern application of essential oils in wellness and self-care routines.

The Renaissance period marked a resurgence in the interest in essential oils in Europe. Alchemists and herbalists began to study the properties of plants more systematically, leading to the distillation techniques that we recognize today. The introduction of steam distillation in the 16th century revolutionized the extraction of essential oils, making them more accessible and pure. This period saw the establishment of essential oils as valuable commodities in trade, expanding their reach and application in perfumery and medicine. The blending of essential oils for aromatic and therapeutic purposes became a respected practice, paving the way for the modern aromatherapy movement.

In the 20th century, the field of aromatherapy gained momentum, particularly through the work of French chemist René-Maurice Gattefossé. His exploration of the therapeutic properties of essential oils led to the recognition of their potential in promoting health and well-being. The modern era has witnessed a growing interest in natural and alternative products, with essential oils being celebrated for their versatility. Today, they are widely used in various applications, including skincare, cleaning solutions, and culinary practices, with an emphasis on their natural origins and holistic benefits.

As society increasingly seeks natural alternatives for health and wellness, essential oils continue to play a significant role. With a rich historical foundation, their applications have expanded into areas such as pet care, meditation, and seasonal support. The ability to craft personalized essential oil blends for various needs has empowered individuals to explore their own aromatic journeys. This ongoing evolution attests to the enduring appeal of essential oils as a means of enhancing life through natural, aromatic solutions, aligning perfectly with the modern desire for sustainable and effective products.

Understanding Essential Oil Extraction

Essential oils are concentrated plant extracts that capture the natural fragrance and therapeutic properties of their source. The extraction process is crucial, as it determines the quality, potency, and characteristics of the essential oil. There are several methods of extraction, with steam distillation and cold pressing being the most common techniques. Steam distillation involves passing steam through plant materials, allowing the volatile compounds to evaporate and then condense back into a liquid. This method is particularly effective for extracting oils from herbs, flowers, and roots, preserving their aromatic and therapeutic qualities.

Cold pressing, on the other hand, is primarily used for citrus fruits. In this method, the outer peel is mechanically pressed to release the essential oil. This technique is favored for its ability to maintain the fresh, zesty scent of citrus oils, making them popular in culinary recipes and natural cleaning solutions. Understanding the extraction method helps consumers choose the right essential oils for their needs, whether for enhancing wellness, creating DIY skincare recipes, or formulating natural cleaning products.

Another extraction method worth noting is solvent extraction, which uses chemical solvents to dissolve the essential oils from plant materials. This technique is often employed for delicate flowers that cannot withstand heat, such as jasmine and rose. Although solvent extraction can yield fragrant oils, the presence of residual solvents can be a concern for those focused on purity and natural products. It is essential for consumers to be aware of the extraction method used to ensure they select high-quality oils, especially for applications such as aromatherapy, skincare, and pet care.

CO2 extraction is a more advanced technique that uses carbon dioxide under high pressure to extract essential oils without the use of heat or solvents. This method produces highly concentrated and pure oils, maintaining the full spectrum of the plant's constituents. CO2-extracted oils are often preferred for wellness applications, as they retain a broader range of therapeutic properties. As consumers become more educated about extraction methods, they can make informed choices that align with their values regarding natural products and holistic health.

In conclusion, understanding essential oil extraction is vital for anyone looking to incorporate these potent plant extracts into their lives. Whether for enhancing relaxation through meditation, supporting seasonal wellness, or crafting unique home fragrance blends, the extraction method impacts the quality and efficacy of the oils. By familiarizing themselves with the various extraction techniques, consumers can better select essential oils that meet their specific needs and contribute to a healthier, more aromatic lifestyle.

The Science Behind Aromatherapy

The science behind aromatherapy is rooted in the understanding of how essential oils interact with the body and mind. Essential oils are concentrated plant extracts that contain volatile compounds, which are responsible for their characteristic fragrances and therapeutic properties. When inhaled, these compounds can influence the limbic system, the part of the brain that governs emotions and memories. This interaction is a key component of how aromatherapy can promote relaxation, alleviate stress, and even enhance mood. The physiological effects of essential oils can be both immediate and profound, making them a valuable tool for those seeking natural alternatives for emotional and physical well-being.

Each essential oil carries its unique profile of chemical compounds, which contribute to its specific benefits. For example, lavender oil is known for its calming properties, thanks to its high levels of linalool and linalyl acetate. These compounds help to reduce anxiety and promote better sleep. Conversely, oils such as peppermint contain menthol and other compounds that can invigorate the mind and improve focus. Understanding these chemical constituents allows users to craft targeted blends that address specific needs, whether for relaxation, energy, or even immune support. This knowledge empowers individuals to create their own personalized aromatherapy experiences based on their unique preferences and requirements.

The application of essential oils extends beyond emotional wellness. In terms of physical health, certain essential oils possess antimicrobial, antifungal, and anti-inflammatory properties, making them useful in natural skincare formulations and cleaning solutions. For instance, tea tree oil is widely recognized for its antiseptic qualities and is often included in DIY skincare recipes to help treat acne and blemishes. Similarly, eucalyptus oil can be a powerful ally in natural cleaning, as it not only disinfects surfaces but also leaves a refreshing scent. By harnessing the science of essential oils, individuals can create effective, natural alternatives to commercial products in their daily routines.

Aromatherapy's benefits also encompass culinary uses, where essential oils can enhance flavors and provide health benefits. Citrus oils, like lemon and orange, can be used sparingly in cooking to infuse dishes with vibrant flavors while also promoting digestion and overall wellness. However, caution is advised in their use, as essential oils are highly concentrated and should be used in moderation. For those interested in pet care, certain essential oils can assist in creating a calming environment for pets or addressing common ailments, although it is crucial to consult with a veterinarian before introducing any new product into an animal's care regimen.

As more people turn to natural solutions for health and wellness, the science behind aromatherapy offers a compelling case for its integration into daily life. Whether for enhancing meditation practices, supporting seasonal allergy relief, or creating home fragrances, essential oils provide a versatile array of options. By understanding the chemical properties and benefits of various oils, individuals can confidently explore the world of aromatherapy, crafting blends that not only elevate their surroundings but also nurture their mind and body.

Chapter 2: Essential Oils for Aromatherapy Blends

The Basics of Aromatherapy

Aromatherapy is a holistic practice that utilizes the fragrant properties of essential oils to promote physical, emotional, and mental well-being. At its core, aromatherapy involves the extraction of essential oils from various plants, including flowers, leaves, stems, and roots, which are then used in various applications such as inhalation, topical application, and diffusion. These essential oils possess unique therapeutic qualities that can enhance mood, alleviate stress, and support overall health. Understanding the basics of aromatherapy is essential for anyone looking to incorporate these natural products into their daily lives.

One of the fundamental principles of aromatherapy is the concept of synergy, where the combined effects of different essential oils can create a more potent impact than when used individually. For instance, blending oils like lavender, known for its calming effects, with eucalyptus, which is often used for respiratory support, can create a powerful blend that promotes relaxation while also addressing seasonal allergies. By experimenting with various combinations, individuals can craft personalized essential oil blends tailored to their specific needs, whether for wellness, relaxation, or even culinary applications.

Essential oils can also be used for DIY skincare recipes, offering a natural alternative to commercial products laden with synthetic ingredients. Oils such as tea tree and frankincense are renowned for their skin-enhancing properties, making them popular choices in homemade beauty formulations. Additionally, essential oils can be seamlessly integrated into natural cleaning solutions, providing not only a fresh scent but also antimicrobial benefits. Oils like lemon and thyme can effectively help sanitize surfaces while imparting a pleasant aroma throughout the home.

The versatility of essential oils extends beyond just personal care and cleaning; they also play a significant role in enhancing wellness and immune support. Certain oils, such as oregano and lemon, are known for their immune-boosting properties, making them valuable additions to daily routines, especially during cold and flu seasons. Furthermore, incorporating essential oils into meditation and relaxation practices can deepen the experience, as scents like cedarwood and chamomile promote tranquility and mindfulness. This holistic approach to wellness can significantly enhance both physical health and emotional balance.

Finally, essential oils can enrich the environment in which we live, offering natural fragrances without the harmful chemicals often found in conventional air fresheners. Using a diffuser to disperse oils like bergamot or ylang-ylang can create a calming atmosphere conducive to relaxation or productivity. In addition, pet owners can explore safe essential oil options that support their furry companions' health and well-being. By understanding the basics of aromatherapy, individuals can effectively harness the power of essential oils to enhance their lives, offering a natural and holistic approach to health, beauty, and home care.

Popular Essential Oils and Their Benefits

Lavender essential oil is one of the most popular and versatile oils used in aromatherapy and skincare. Renowned for its calming and soothing properties, lavender can help alleviate stress, anxiety, and promote restful sleep. In DIY skincare, it serves as an excellent addition to moisturizers and serums, thanks to its anti-inflammatory and antiseptic qualities. Furthermore, lavender oil can be incorporated into natural cleaning solutions for its pleasant aroma and antimicrobial effects, making it a favorite for those seeking a holistic approach to home care.

Tea tree essential oil is another powerhouse in the world of natural remedies, often celebrated for its potent antibacterial and antifungal properties. It is a staple in DIY skincare recipes, particularly for acne treatment and soothing skin irritations. Beyond skincare, tea tree oil can be used in natural cleaning products, effectively disinfecting surfaces and purifying the air. Its versatility also extends to pet care, as it can be safely diluted and used to combat pests, making it an excellent choice for pet owners looking for natural solutions.

Peppermint essential oil offers refreshing and invigorating benefits, making it a favorite for both culinary uses and wellness support. In the kitchen, a drop of peppermint oil can elevate desserts and beverages, adding a burst of flavor. In terms of wellness, peppermint is known to aid digestion and relieve headaches, making it a valuable addition to aromatherapy blends. Many individuals also use peppermint oil in homemade hair care treatments, as it promotes scalp health and stimulates hair growth, providing a natural alternative for those seeking hair care solutions.

Eucalyptus essential oil is particularly valued for its respiratory benefits, making it a go-to for seasonal allergies and immune support. Its strong, fresh scent helps clear nasal passages and can be particularly effective in diffusers during cold and flu season. Eucalyptus oil can be blended with other essential oils to create calming and rejuvenating blends for meditation and relaxation practices. Additionally, it can be included in natural cleaning solutions, providing a refreshing aroma while also acting as a disinfectant.

Finally, citrus essential oils, such as lemon and orange, are celebrated for their uplifting and energizing properties. These oils are commonly used in home fragrance diffusers, creating a bright and cheerful atmosphere. In culinary recipes, citrus oils add a zesty flavor, enhancing both sweet and savory dishes. Their antibacterial properties also make them an excellent choice for natural cleaning solutions, helping to purify and freshen the home. For those looking to incorporate essential oils into their daily routine, citrus oils provide a delightful and versatile option that supports both wellness and a pleasant living environment.

Creating Your First Aromatherapy Blend

Creating your first aromatherapy blend can be an exciting and fulfilling experience, especially as you explore the myriad benefits that essential oils can offer for both mind and body. To begin, it is important to understand the basic components of essential oil blending. Essential oils are highly concentrated plant extracts, each with unique properties and aromas. When creating a blend, consider the purpose of your blend—whether it's for relaxation, uplifting energy, or even supporting your immune system. Start by selecting a few essential oils that resonate with your goals, ensuring they complement each other both in scent and therapeutic benefits.

Before you start measuring and mixing, familiarize yourself with the oils you've chosen. Research their individual properties, safety precautions, and any contraindications, especially if you plan to use them on your skin or around pets. For a basic blend, choose one or two top notes, which are typically fresh and uplifting scents like lemon or peppermint; one middle note, often more balanced and soothing, such as lavender or geranium; and one base note, which adds depth and richness, like sandalwood or patchouli. This layered approach not only creates a harmonious fragrance but also enhances the therapeutic properties of the blend.

When you're ready to create your blend, use a glass dropper to measure each essential oil accurately. Start with small quantities, such as five to ten drops of each oil, and mix them in a glass bottle. This allows you to experiment without wasting your precious oils. As you mix, take note of the scent and how it evolves. You may need to adjust the ratios, adding more of a particular oil to achieve your desired aroma or therapeutic effect. Keep in mind that essential oils can be potent, so it's often wise to err on the side of caution and build up the scent gradually.

Once you are satisfied with your blend, it's crucial to dilute it properly, especially if you plan to use it for skincare or massage. A typical dilution ratio for topical application is 2-3% essential oil to carrier oil, such as jojoba, sweet almond, or coconut oil. For instance, if you have a 10ml bottle, adding around 6-9 drops of your essential oil blend to the carrier oil will create a safe mixture for application on the skin. Always perform a patch test before using it extensively to ensure there are no adverse reactions.

Finally, don't forget to label your blend with the ingredients and the date you created it. This not only helps you keep track of your creations but also allows you to refine your technique over time. Remember that creating aromatherapy blends is an art as much as it is a science, so embrace the process and be open to adjustments in future blends. With practice, you will develop your intuition and knowledge, making the crafting of essential oil blends a rewarding and enriching experience that enhances your wellness journey.

Chapter 3: DIY Essential Oil Skincare Recipes

Essential Oils for Different Skin Types

Essential oils have gained popularity not only for their aromatic benefits but also for their potential in skincare. Understanding the unique needs of different skin types is crucial when selecting essential oils for topical applications. Each skin type—whether oily, dry, sensitive, or combination—has specific characteristics that can be addressed through tailored essential oil blends. By selecting the right oils, individuals can enhance their skincare routines, promoting healthier skin while embracing natural alternatives.

For oily skin, essential oils that possess astringent and antibacterial properties can be particularly beneficial. Oils such as tea tree, lavender, and rosemary are excellent choices, as they help to reduce excess oil production and combat acne-causing bacteria. A simple DIY blend can be created using a carrier oil like jojoba, which mimics the skin's natural sebum, combined with a few drops of tea tree oil and lavender. This blend not only helps control oiliness but also soothes inflammation and promotes healing.

Dry skin, on the other hand, requires oils that provide deep hydration and nourishment. Essential oils like frankincense, geranium, and sandalwood are known for their moisturizing properties. A DIY recipe for dry skin might include a base of sweet almond oil, combined with drops of geranium and frankincense. This blend can help lock in moisture, improve skin elasticity, and reduce the appearance of fine lines. Incorporating these oils into a nightly skincare routine can provide the hydration that dry skin craves.

Sensitive skin requires a gentle approach, and essential oils that are calming and anti-inflammatory are ideal. Oils such as chamomile, lavender, and helichrysum can help soothe irritation and redness. A calming blend could consist of a light carrier oil like fractionated coconut oil mixed with chamomile and lavender. This combination not only alleviates discomfort but also promotes a sense of peace, making it suitable for those who experience skin sensitivity or conditions like rosacea.

Combination skin presents a unique challenge, as it encompasses both oily and dry areas. Essential oils that balance out these opposing needs are essential. Oils like ylang-ylang and bergamot can help to regulate oil production while providing moisture to drier patches. A balanced blend might include a carrier oil such as grapeseed oil, combined with ylang-ylang and bergamot. This versatile formulation can help achieve a more harmonious complexion, addressing the varying needs of combination skin effectively. By understanding the properties of essential oils and their alignment with different skin types, individuals can craft personalized skincare solutions that nurture and enhance their natural beauty.

Recipes for Facial Blends

Creating your own facial blends using essential oils offers a personalized approach to skincare, allowing you to cater to your specific skin type and concerns. Essential oils not only provide aromatic benefits but also possess unique therapeutic properties that can enhance your skincare routine. To begin, it's crucial to understand the characteristics of different oils. For instance, lavender is known for its calming effects and can help soothe irritated skin, while tea tree oil is renowned for its antibacterial properties, making it a great choice for acne-prone skin.

For a nourishing facial blend ideal for dry skin, combine five drops of sandalwood oil, four drops of frankincense oil, and three drops of geranium oil with a carrier oil such as jojoba or sweet almond oil. This blend not only hydrates and revitalizes the skin but also promotes a sense of grounding and tranquility. Apply this mixture after cleansing your face to lock in moisture and provide essential nutrients. Additionally, the soothing aroma of sandalwood can create a calming atmosphere during your skincare routine.

If you're targeting oily or combination skin, consider crafting a blend with three drops of rosemary oil, three drops of lemon oil, and two drops of lavender oil. Mix these oils with a base of grapeseed oil, which is lightweight and balances oily skin. This combination helps to regulate sebum production while offering a refreshing scent that can uplift your mood. Apply it in the morning and evening to help maintain a clear complexion and enjoy the invigorating properties of lemon oil.

For those dealing with signs of aging, a rejuvenating facial blend can be made using four drops of helichrysum oil, three drops of rose oil, and two drops of patchouli oil, combined with a carrier oil like argan oil. Known for its regenerative properties, helichrysum oil can promote skin elasticity, while rose oil provides deep hydration and a luxurious scent. Apply this blend gently around the eyes and on the forehead to target fine lines and wrinkles, creating a spa-like experience at home.

Lastly, a soothing facial blend for sensitive skin can be created with four drops of chamomile oil, three drops of lavender oil, and two drops of geranium oil, mixed with aloe vera gel or a gentle carrier oil. This combination helps to calm redness and irritation while promoting healing. Use this blend as a relaxing facial treatment, especially after a long day or exposure to environmental stressors. Incorporating these essential oil blends into your skincare routine not only enhances your skin's health but also provides a moment of self-care and relaxation.

Body Care Recipes with Essential Oils

Body care recipes utilizing essential oils offer a natural and effective way to enhance your skincare routine while promoting overall wellness. These recipes harness the therapeutic properties of essential oils, which not only provide delightful fragrances but also contribute to skin health and emotional balance. By incorporating essential oils into your body care regimen, you can create personalized products that cater to your specific needs, from moisturizing lotions to soothing balms.

To create a nourishing body lotion, consider blending coconut oil, shea butter, and your choice of essential oils such as lavender or tea tree oil. Start by melting equal parts of coconut oil and shea butter in a double boiler. Once melted, remove from heat and allow to cool slightly before adding around 10-15 drops of your selected essential oil. Lavender is known for its calming properties, making it perfect for relaxation, while tea tree oil offers antiseptic benefits. Whip the mixture until it reaches a creamy consistency and store it in a glass jar for easy use.

Another excellent body care recipe is a rejuvenating scrub that can exfoliate and hydrate your skin. Combine brown sugar or sea salt with a carrier oil like olive or almond oil, and add essential oils such as peppermint or eucalyptus for a refreshing twist. The sugar or salt acts as an exfoliant, while the carrier oil moisturizes the skin. Adding a few drops of peppermint essential oil not only invigorates your senses but also helps improve circulation, making it ideal for an energizing morning routine.

For those seeking natural alternatives to commercial deodorants, a simple recipe can be crafted using baking soda, cornstarch, coconut oil, and essential oils like lemon or rosemary. Mix equal parts of baking soda and cornstarch in a bowl, then add melted coconut oil until you achieve a paste-like consistency. Incorporate 10 drops of your chosen essential oil for its antibacterial properties and pleasant fragrance. This natural deodorant can help neutralize odors while allowing your skin to breathe, a preferable option for many looking to avoid synthetic ingredients.

In addition to skincare, essential oils can play a significant role in hair care. A revitalizing hair mask can be made by combining avocado or coconut oil with essential oils like rosemary or lavender.

Apply the mixture to your hair, focusing on the scalp, and leave it on for 30 minutes before washing it out. Rosemary oil is renowned for stimulating hair growth, while lavender can soothe the scalp and reduce dandruff. Incorporating these recipes into your routine not only nourishes your body but also aligns with a holistic approach to self-care, utilizing the power of nature for your health and well-being.

Chapter 4: Essential Oils for Natural Cleaning Solutions

Benefits of Using Essential Oils for Cleaning

The use of essential oils for cleaning provides a natural alternative to traditional chemical-based products, which often contain harsh ingredients that can be harmful to both health and the environment. Essential oils, derived from plants, offer potent antibacterial, antifungal, and antiviral properties that make them effective agents for sanitizing and deodorizing various surfaces in the home. By opting for essential oils, individuals can create a cleaner environment that is safer for their families, pets, and the planet.

One of the key benefits of using essential oils for cleaning is their ability to purify the air. Many essential oils, such as tea tree and eucalyptus, have natural properties that help eliminate airborne pathogens and allergens. When diffused or added to cleaning solutions, these oils can improve indoor air quality, making them particularly beneficial for those with respiratory issues, allergies, or sensitivities. This aspect of essential oils not only enhances the cleanliness of the home but also contributes to overall wellness and comfort.

In addition to their health benefits, essential oils also introduce delightful fragrances into cleaning routines. Unlike synthetic fragrances that can trigger allergies or irritate the senses, essential oils offer a range of natural scents that can elevate mood and promote feelings of relaxation and happiness. Citrus oils like lemon and orange can invigorate and energize, while lavender can provide a calming atmosphere. This makes cleaning not just a chore, but an aromatic experience that can enhance mental well-being.

Furthermore, essential oils are incredibly versatile and can be incorporated into various DIY cleaning recipes. From all-purpose sprays to laundry detergents, the possibilities for blending essential oils are vast. This flexibility allows individuals to customize their cleaning solutions according to personal preferences and specific cleaning needs. For those interested in sustainability, using essential oils reduces reliance on single-use plastic containers often found in commercial cleaning products, contributing to a more eco-conscious lifestyle.

Finally, integrating essential oils into cleaning routines aligns with a broader movement toward holistic wellness. The ritual of cleaning with essential oils can transform the mundane task into a mindful practice, encouraging individuals to focus on their intention and connection to their environment. This approach not only fosters a cleaner home but also promotes a sense of balance and harmony, making essential oils an invaluable tool for those seeking natural alternatives in their daily lives.

Recipes for All-Purpose Cleaners

Creating your own all-purpose cleaners with essential oils not only provides an effective cleaning solution but also infuses your home with delightful aromas. These natural alternatives are free from harsh chemicals, making them safe for your family and pets. This subchapter presents several recipes for all-purpose cleaners that harness the power of essential oils, allowing you to maintain a clean and fresh environment while promoting wellness through aromatic properties.

A basic all-purpose cleaner can be made using just a few simple ingredients. Combine one cup of white vinegar with one cup of water in a spray bottle. To this mixture, add 20 drops of your favorite essential oils, such as lemon for its antibacterial properties or lavender for its calming scent. Shake well before use. This cleaner is effective on countertops, bathroom surfaces, and even kitchen appliances. The vinegar acts as a natural disinfectant, while the essential oils enhance the cleaning power and provide a pleasant fragrance.

For a more robust cleaning solution that tackles tough stains and grime, consider a recipe with baking soda. In a bowl, mix one cup of baking soda with half a cup of liquid castile soap and 15 drops of tea tree oil, known for its antifungal and antibacterial characteristics. Slowly add water until you achieve a paste-like consistency. Apply this mixture to stubborn areas, let it sit for a few minutes, and then scrub away. This paste not only cleans effectively but also leaves a refreshing scent in its wake.

If you prefer a citrusy aroma, try a citrus-infused all-purpose cleaner. In a quart-sized jar, combine peels from oranges, lemons, or limes with a cup of vinegar. Let this mixture sit for at least two weeks to allow the oils in the peels to infuse the vinegar. After the infusion period, strain the liquid into a spray bottle, diluting it with an equal amount of water. Add 10 drops of essential oil, such as grapefruit or bergamot, for an extra boost. This cleaner is particularly effective for cutting through grease and leaving surfaces sparkling.

Lastly, for a fresh scent that promotes relaxation, create a lavender and rosemary cleaner. Mix two cups of water, half a cup of vinegar, and 10 drops each of lavender and rosemary essential oils in a spray bottle. This combination not only cleans effectively but also transforms your cleaning routine into a calming experience. Use this cleaner on surfaces where you want to evoke a sense of tranquility, such as in bedrooms or living areas. With these recipes, you can enjoy a naturally clean home infused with the therapeutic benefits of essential oils.

Specific Solutions for Common Household Issues

In the realm of household issues, essential oils offer a myriad of specific solutions that cater to various needs. For those seeking natural alternatives, essential oils serve as effective remedies for common problems, from cleaning surfaces to enhancing personal care routines. Each essential oil possesses unique properties that can be harnessed to create blends tailored for individual concerns. This subchapter explores how to utilize essential oils to address specific household issues, promoting wellness and harmony within the home environment.

One common household issue is the presence of unpleasant odors. Essential oils such as lemon, lavender, and eucalyptus can be utilized in home fragrance diffusers to purify the air and create a soothing atmosphere. A simple blend of these oils not only masks odors but also offers antibacterial properties that help eliminate the source of unpleasant smells. For a natural air freshener, combine these essential oils with water in a spray bottle to create a refreshing mist that can be used throughout the home, ensuring a clean and inviting environment.

Another area where essential oils shine is in skincare. DIY essential oil skincare recipes using oils like tea tree, frankincense, and rose can address a variety of skin concerns, including acne, aging, and dryness. By combining these oils with carrier oils such as jojoba or coconut oil, individuals can create personalized serums and moisturizers that nourish the skin without harsh chemicals. This approach not only promotes healthier skin but also allows for a more mindful self-care routine, reinforcing the importance of using natural products in daily life.

For those interested in maintaining a clean home, essential oils can be powerful allies in natural cleaning solutions. Oils such as tea tree, lemon, and peppermint possess antimicrobial properties that make them ideal for disinfecting surfaces. A simple all-purpose cleaner can be made by combining vinegar, water, and a few drops of these essential oils. This not only ensures a germ-free environment but also allows homeowners to avoid the toxic chemicals often found in commercial cleaning products, aligning with a more holistic approach to home care.

Essential oils also play a significant role in wellness and immune support, especially during seasonal changes. Oils like oregano, eucalyptus, and lavender can be diffused to support respiratory health and enhance mood. In addition, these oils can be incorporated into culinary recipes, providing both flavor and health benefits. For example, adding a drop of oregano oil to soups or stews can boost the dish's nutritional profile while supporting the immune system. Furthermore, essential oils can be utilized in pet care and relaxation practices, ensuring that every member of the household reaps the benefits of nature's offerings. By integrating essential oils into various aspects of home life, individuals can create a sanctuary that nurtures both body and mind.

Chapter 5: Essential Oils for Wellness and Immune Support

Essential Oils to Boost Immunity

Essential oils have gained recognition for their potential to support and enhance the immune system, offering a natural alternative to conventional remedies. Many essential oils possess antimicrobial, antiviral, and anti-inflammatory properties, making them valuable allies in promoting overall wellness. By incorporating these oils into your daily routine, you can create a holistic approach to maintaining your health, particularly during cold and flu seasons or times of increased stress.

Among the most effective essential oils for boosting immunity is eucalyptus oil. Renowned for its ability to clear the respiratory tract, eucalyptus also boasts properties that can help fight infections. This oil can be used in diffusers or added to steam inhalation therapies to support respiratory health. Another powerful oil is tea tree oil, which is celebrated for its antiseptic qualities. It can be incorporated into DIY skincare recipes, providing a natural solution for blemishes and skin irritations while also enhancing your immune defenses.

Lemon essential oil is another excellent choice for immune support, thanks to its high vitamin C content and antioxidant properties. It can be easily added to culinary recipes or used in homemade cleaning solutions, combining delightful fragrance with immune-boosting benefits. In aromatherapy, lemon oil can uplift the spirit and promote a sense of well-being, making it a versatile addition to any wellness routine. Incorporating it into your daily rituals can provide both physical and emotional support.

Oregano oil is often considered a powerhouse for immune health, known for its potent antiviral and antibacterial properties. This oil can be used in culinary dishes, providing flavor while delivering health benefits. For those engaged in pet care, oregano oil can also be diluted and used to support your furry friends' immune systems, though it's crucial to ensure that oils are safe for animal use. Always consult with a veterinarian to determine the best practices for incorporating essential oils into your pets' routines.

Finally, incorporating essential oils like lavender and rosemary into your meditation and relaxation practices can further enhance your immune response. Lavender is known for its calming effects, which can reduce stress and promote better sleep—two critical factors for a healthy immune system. Rosemary, on the other hand, is believed to stimulate circulation and enhance cognitive function. By creating personalized blends using these oils, you can cultivate a serene environment that nurtures both mind and body, ultimately leading to improved immunity and wellness.

Blends for Stress Relief and Relaxation

Blends for stress relief and relaxation play a crucial role in the world of aromatherapy, offering a natural alternative to conventional methods of managing stress. Essential oils possess unique properties that can help soothe the mind and body, promoting a sense of calm and well-being. By carefully selecting and combining these oils, individuals can create personalized blends that cater to their specific needs. Lavender, chamomile, and bergamot are among the most popular essential oils known for their relaxing effects, making them ideal candidates for crafting stress-relief formulations.

When formulating a stress-relief blend, it is essential to consider the various methods of application. Diffusion is one of the most effective ways to experience the benefits of essential oils. Simply adding a few drops of your chosen blend to a diffuser can fill your space with calming aromas that help reduce anxiety and create a serene environment. Alternatively, creating a rollerball blend for topical application allows for convenient use throughout the day. A mix of calming oils diluted in a carrier oil can be applied to pulse points or the back of the neck, providing on-the-go relief from stress.

In addition to their aromatic qualities, essential oils can also enhance skincare routines, promoting relaxation during self-care rituals. Blending oils like ylang-ylang or sandalwood with a base of coconut or jojoba oil creates a soothing massage oil that not only nourishes the skin but also provides a calming effect. Incorporating these blends into a lotion or cream can further enhance the experience, allowing the user to indulge in a fragrant, stress-relieving moment. This approach integrates wellness and relaxation into daily routines, making self-care a priority.

For those seeking an all-encompassing approach to stress relief, incorporating essential oils into cleaning solutions can create a peaceful atmosphere while maintaining a healthy home environment. Oils such as lemon and eucalyptus not only purify the air but also elevate the mood during routine cleaning tasks. By adding a few drops of calming essential oils to homemade cleaning products, individuals can transform mundane chores into uplifting experiences, fostering a sense of tranquility throughout the home.

Lastly, essential oils can be a powerful addition to meditation and mindfulness practices. Creating a calming atmosphere is vital for enhancing focus and relaxation during these sessions. Blends featuring frankincense, cedarwood, or patchouli can ground the mind and assist in achieving a deeper state of meditation. By diffusing these oils or using them in personal inhalers, individuals can cultivate a sacred space that promotes relaxation and inner peace. These aromatic blends not only support mental clarity and emotional balance but also contribute to a holistic approach to wellness that resonates with those seeking natural alternatives.

Seasonal Support with Essential Oils

Seasonal changes can bring about a variety of challenges, from allergies to skin issues, making it essential to equip ourselves with natural solutions. Essential oils offer a versatile approach to support both mind and body during these transitional times. By understanding the properties of specific oils, you can create blends that not only enhance your well-being but also address seasonal concerns effectively. This section will explore how you can utilize essential oils for a range of seasonal support needs.

For those suffering from seasonal allergies, certain essential oils can provide relief by reducing inflammation and promoting respiratory health. Oils such as lavender, eucalyptus, and peppermint are known for their soothing properties. Diffusing these oils in your home can help clear your airways and create a calm atmosphere. Additionally, incorporating these oils into personal inhalers or topical blends can offer on-the-go relief, making it easier to manage symptoms throughout the day.

As the seasons change, so too can our skin's needs. Essential oils like tea tree, frankincense, and chamomile can be beneficial in DIY skincare recipes to combat dryness or irritation. Creating a nourishing facial serum or a soothing body lotion with these oils can help maintain your skin's health and hydration. Remember to always dilute essential oils in a carrier oil before applying them to your skin to avoid irritation, ensuring a safe and pleasant experience.

In the realm of wellness and immune support, essential oils can play a significant role. Blends containing oils such as oregano, lemon, and thyme can bolster your immune system, particularly during the colder months when colds and flu are prevalent. It is easy to incorporate these oils into your daily routine, whether through inhalation, topical application, or even in culinary recipes. Adding a few drops of lemon or oregano to your meals not only enhances flavor but also boosts your health.

Cleaning your home effectively while maintaining a natural approach is another area where essential oils shine. Oils like tea tree, lemon, and lavender possess antimicrobial properties, making them perfect for natural cleaning solutions. By creating your own cleaning sprays or surface wipes with these oils, you can ensure that your living environment remains fresh and free from harmful chemicals.

This not only promotes a cleaner home but also contributes to a healthier atmosphere for you and your family.

Finally, essential oils can enhance your meditation and relaxation practices, which are especially important during seasonal transitions. Oils such as sandalwood, bergamot, and ylang-ylang can promote tranquility and peace of mind. Utilizing these oils in a diffuser during meditation or incorporating them into a calming bath can create a serene environment, allowing you to fully embrace the changing seasons with a centered and relaxed mindset. By harnessing the power of essential oils, you can navigate seasonal shifts with grace and wellness.

Chapter 6: Essential Oils in Culinary Recipes

Cooking with Essential Oils: Safety and Guidelines

Cooking with essential oils can open up a world of flavor and wellness, but it is essential to approach this practice with care and knowledge. Not all essential oils are safe for consumption, and even those that are must be used with caution. To ensure a positive and beneficial experience, it's crucial to understand which oils are safe to use in culinary applications, how to measure them properly, and the best practices for incorporating them into your recipes.

When selecting essential oils for cooking, it's important to choose high-quality, food-grade oils. Not all essential oils are created equal; some may contain additives or impurities that can be harmful if ingested. Look for oils that are labeled as safe for culinary use. Common essential oils that are typically safe for consumption include lemon, peppermint, and lavender, among others. Always verify the source and ensure that the oils are pure and derived from reputable suppliers.

Safety is paramount when using essential oils in cooking. They are highly concentrated substances, and a little goes a long way. It is advisable to start with just one drop of essential oil in your dish and gradually increase the amount to taste. Remember that the flavor of essential oils can intensify over time, so be cautious when adding them to recipes. Additionally, some oils may interact with medications or have contraindications for certain health conditions, so consulting with a healthcare professional before introducing them into your diet is wise.

In addition to culinary uses, essential oils can enhance your overall well-being when incorporated into DIY skincare, natural cleaning solutions, and home fragrance diffusers. When creating skin care products or cleaning solutions, always perform a patch test to check for skin sensitivities. For essential oils used in meditation and relaxation, consider blending them with carrier oils or using them in diffusers to create a calming atmosphere. This ensures that you benefit from their therapeutic properties while minimizing any potential adverse reactions.

Finally, when using essential oils for pet care, it's vital to conduct thorough research, as some oils can be toxic to animals. Always consult a veterinarian before using essential oils around pets. When it comes to seasonal allergies, oils like eucalyptus and tea tree may provide relief, but again, approach with caution and awareness of individual sensitivities. By following these safety guidelines and understanding the proper use of essential oils, you can effectively incorporate them into your cooking and self-care routine, enhancing both flavor and wellness in your life.

Flavorful Essential Oil Infusions

In the realm of natural products, essential oils have emerged as versatile tools for enhancing well-being and creating harmonious environments. Flavorful essential oil infusions offer a unique way to incorporate these aromatic compounds into daily life, enriching not only the sensory experience but also providing various health benefits. By understanding how to craft these infusions, individuals can seamlessly integrate essential oils into aromatherapy blends, DIY skincare recipes, and even culinary creations.

When infusing essential oils, the quality of the oils and the method of infusion are paramount. Cold-pressed or steam-distilled essential oils retain their therapeutic properties and are ideal for creating blends. For skincare, combining essential oils with carrier oils such as jojoba or sweet almond oil can enhance their effectiveness while providing moisture. Specific blends can target various skin concerns; for instance, lavender and tea tree oil can be infused to create a soothing, antibacterial serum that rejuvenates tired skin.

Incorporating essential oils into cleaning solutions not only elevates the sensory experience but also harnesses their natural antibacterial and antiviral properties. Citrus oils like lemon and orange, when infused into homemade cleaning sprays, can provide a refreshing scent while effectively cutting through grease and grime. Infusing oils into all-natural cleaning recipes makes the process safer for both the environment and the household, minimizing exposure to harsh chemicals often found in commercial products.

The culinary world also stands to benefit from essential oil infusions, providing a novel approach to flavoring dishes. Oils such as peppermint, lemon, and basil can be infused into oils or vinegars, allowing for unique flavor profiles that enhance meals. When using essential oils in cooking, it is crucial to consider their potency; a drop or two can go a long way. This method not only adds an aromatic touch but also brings the potential health benefits of the oils into the dining experience, supporting wellness and immune function.

Lastly, flavorful essential oil infusions can be a delightful addition to pet care and home fragrance. Infusing oils like chamomile or cedarwood into pet grooming products can promote relaxation and comfort, benefiting both pets and their owners. For home fragrance diffusers, essential oils such as eucalyptus or lavender can create a calming atmosphere, perfect for meditation and relaxation practices. By exploring the many applications of flavorful essential oil infusions, individuals can tap into the power of nature, enhancing their lifestyles with natural and aromatic solutions.

Recipes for Savory Dishes and Desserts

In the realm of culinary creativity, essential oils can transform ordinary dishes and desserts into aromatic experiences that tantalize the senses. This subchapter presents a collection of savory recipes and sweet treats that incorporate essential oils, allowing you to explore new flavor dimensions while enjoying the health benefits they offer. Whether you're crafting a comforting meal or a delightful dessert, these recipes utilize essential oils known for their culinary properties, enhancing both taste and wellness.

For a savory delight, consider preparing a rosemary-infused roasted vegetable medley. Begin by selecting seasonal vegetables such as zucchini, bell peppers, and carrots. Toss them in olive oil and sprinkle with a drop or two of rosemary essential oil, along with salt and pepper. Roast them at 400°F until they are tender and caramelized. The rosemary not only adds a fragrant herbaceous note but also contributes antioxidant properties, making this dish both nutritious and flavorful. Pair it with a protein of your choice for a well-rounded meal.

Another exciting savory option is lemon-infused quinoa salad. Cook quinoa according to package instructions, then let it cool. In a bowl, combine the quinoa with diced cucumbers, cherry tomatoes, and red onion. For the dressing, whisk together olive oil, lemon juice, and a drop of lemon essential oil. This bright and refreshing dish is perfect for summer gatherings or as a light lunch. The lemon essential oil enhances the flavor profile while providing a boost of vitamin C, supporting your immune system.

Moving on to desserts, essential oils can elevate your sweet creations. A classic vanilla essential oil chocolate mousse is both easy to make and indulgent. Melt dark chocolate and let it cool slightly. Whip together heavy cream and gently fold in the cooled chocolate. Add a drop of vanilla essential oil for depth of flavor. Chill until set, then serve with fresh berries. The aromatic richness of vanilla enhances the dessert's appeal, while its calming properties can aid in relaxation, making it a perfect end to a meal.

Another delightful dessert to try is an orange essential oil-infused panna cotta. Combine cream, sugar, and gelatin, heating until dissolved. Once cooled slightly, add a few drops of orange essential oil and pour into molds. Chill until set, and serve with a berry compote. The bright citrus notes from the orange essential oil bring a refreshing zing to the creamy texture, creating a dessert that is both elegant and healthful, as orange oil is known for its uplifting and invigorating properties.

Incorporating essential oils into your cooking not only enhances flavors but also promotes wellness. By experimenting with these recipes, you can discover the versatility of essential oils in the kitchen, providing both savory and sweet options that cater to a range of tastes and dietary preferences. Whether you're hosting a dinner party or enjoying a quiet evening at home, these dishes will elevate your culinary experience and support your journey toward a more natural lifestyle.

Chapter 7: Essential Oils for Pet Care

Safe Essential Oils for Pets

When considering the use of essential oils around pets, it is crucial to understand which oils are safe and how to use them properly. Many essential oils can be beneficial for pets, aiding in relaxation, skin care, and even natural pest control. However, not all essential oils are safe for animal companions; some can be toxic or irritating. Therefore, it is essential to educate yourself about which oils are safe, how to dilute them, and the appropriate methods of application.

Lavender and chamomile are two of the most widely regarded safe essential oils for pets. Lavender oil, known for its calming properties, can help reduce anxiety in both dogs and cats. A few drops diluted in a carrier oil can be massaged into a pet's skin or added to a diffuser to create a soothing environment. Chamomile is similarly beneficial, providing calming effects and helping to ease digestive issues in pets. Care should be taken to use high-quality, pure essential oils, as synthetic fragrances can be harmful.

Citrus oils, while pleasant for humans, can be problematic for some pets. Dogs may tolerate certain citrus oils, such as sweet orange, when properly diluted, but they can be irritating to cats and should be avoided around them. Always perform a patch test on a small area of your pet's skin when introducing a new essential oil. Monitor them for any adverse reactions, such as redness or excessive scratching, to ensure their safety.

Incorporating essential oils into your pet care routine can also extend to natural cleaning solutions. Essential oils such as eucalyptus and tea tree can be effective in homemade cleaners, but their use around pets should be approached with caution. When using these oils, ensure that your pets are kept away during the cleaning process, and allow areas to dry completely before they return. This practice minimizes the risk of exposure to any potentially harmful residues.

Lastly, when using essential oils for pet care, moderation is key. Always consult with a veterinarian familiar with essential oils to tailor their use to your specific pet's needs. By being informed and cautious, you can safely enjoy the benefits of essential oils while providing a nurturing environment for your furry friends. The right approach can enhance your pet's wellness and create a harmonious atmosphere in your home.

Blends for Pet Anxiety and Relaxation

Blends for pet anxiety and relaxation can play a significant role in enhancing the well-being of our furry companions. Just like humans, pets can experience stress and anxiety from various situations, including loud noises, changes in their environment, or separation from their owners. Essential oils offer a natural approach to help soothe these feelings, fostering a calm atmosphere. When creating blends for pets, it is essential to choose pet-safe oils and to understand the proper dilution ratios to ensure safety and efficacy.

Lavender essential oil is one of the most popular choices for calming anxious pets. Its gentle aroma has been shown to reduce stress and promote relaxation. When blended with other soothing oils like chamomile or bergamot, it can create a powerful calming effect. A simple blend for your pet could include three drops of lavender oil, two drops of chamomile oil, and one drop of bergamot oil. This mixture can be diluted with a carrier oil, such as coconut or jojoba oil, before applying it to a pet's collar or using it in a diffuser in their relaxation space.

Another effective blend incorporates vetiver and ylang-ylang. Vetiver is known for its grounding properties, while ylang-ylang can help alleviate feelings of tension. A recommended blend could consist of two drops of vetiver, two drops of ylang-ylang, and one drop of frankincense. This combination not only calms the mind but also promotes a sense of security. As with any essential oil application, it is crucial to monitor your pet's response and ensure they are comfortable with the scent.

For pets that may be particularly sensitive to scent, a simple blend of sweet orange and cedarwood can be beneficial. Sweet orange offers uplifting properties that can combat feelings of sadness, while cedarwood provides a grounding and woodsy aroma that promotes tranquility. This blend can be made with three drops of sweet orange and two drops of cedarwood, diluted in a carrier oil or used in a diffuser. The uplifting yet calming nature of this blend can create a comforting environment, especially during stressful situations such as thunderstorms or fireworks.

Lastly, incorporating essential oils into your pet care routine can also extend to DIY sprays for calming their space. A spray made from a blend of lavender and distilled water can serve as a natural room spray to help create a peaceful environment. The recommended ratio is about ten drops of lavender essential oil per four ounces of water. This can be lightly misted in areas where your pet spends time, promoting relaxation and reducing anxiety. By thoughtfully crafting essential oil blends for anxiety and relaxation, pet owners can enhance their pets' quality of life through natural and soothing methods.

Natural Solutions for Common Pet Issues

Pet owners often seek natural and holistic approaches to address common issues their furry companions face. Essential oils can serve as valuable tools in promoting the health and well-being of pets when used correctly. This subchapter explores several essential oils that can help with common pet problems, such as anxiety, skin irritations, and natural pest control.

Anxiety is a prevalent issue among pets, particularly during stressful situations like thunderstorms or fireworks. Lavender essential oil is widely recognized for its calming properties and can be an excellent choice for anxious pets. Diffusing lavender in the home or applying a diluted blend to a pet's collar can create a soothing atmosphere. Additionally, chamomile oil may help to relax pets and promote a sense of peace, making it another option for those looking to ease their animals' anxiety.

Skin irritations and allergies are common complaints in pets, often resulting from environmental factors or dietary sensitivities. Essential oils like tea tree and frankincense can be beneficial for soothing irritated skin and promoting healing. When diluted with a carrier oil, these essential oils can be gently massaged into affected areas to provide relief. Moreover, incorporating soothing oils such as geranium can help reduce inflammation and balance the skin's natural barrier, offering further support to pets suffering from dermatological issues.

Natural pest control is another area where essential oils can play a significant role. Many oils possess insect-repelling properties that can help keep pests at bay without the use of harsh chemicals. For instance, peppermint and cedarwood oils are known for their ability to deter fleas and ticks. A diluted spray made with these oils can be applied to pet bedding and living areas, creating a protective environment for pets. It's crucial, however, to ensure any essential oils used are safe and suitable for specific animals, as some oils can be harmful to pets.

Finally, incorporating essential oils into a pet's wellness routine can enhance their overall health and immunity. Oils like eucalyptus and lemon can support respiratory health and boost the immune system. These oils can be diffused in the home or added to homemade pet treats in small, safe quantities. It's essential to consult a veterinarian familiar with essential oils to ensure that the chosen oils are appropriate for the specific pet, as individual sensitivities and health conditions may vary.

In conclusion, essential oils offer a range of natural solutions for addressing common pet issues. From calming anxious pets to soothing skin irritations and providing natural pest control, these oils can enhance the quality of life for many animals. As with any natural remedy, it is vital to use essential oils with caution, ensuring they are properly diluted and safe for the specific needs of each pet. By integrating these natural solutions, pet owners can foster a healthier and more harmonious environment for their beloved companions.

Chapter 8: Essential Oils for Meditation and Relaxation

Creating a Calm Space with Essential Oils

Creating a calm space with essential oils involves understanding the unique properties of various oils and how they can influence our environment and well-being. When looking to establish tranquility in your home, selecting the right essential oils is crucial. Popular options for promoting calmness include lavender, chamomile, and bergamot, which are known for their soothing and relaxing qualities. Incorporating these oils into your space can help alleviate stress, reduce anxiety, and create an atmosphere conducive to relaxation and meditation.

One effective way to utilize essential oils for creating a calm environment is through diffusion. Using an essential oil diffuser allows the oils to disperse into the air, filling the room with their therapeutic aromas. For a calming blend, consider combining lavender oil with sweet orange or cedarwood. This combination not only enhances relaxation but also provides a comforting and inviting ambiance. Diffusing these oils during meditation or yoga sessions can deepen your practice, helping to center your mind and promote a sense of peace.

In addition to diffusion, essential oils can be integrated into your skincare routine to enhance relaxation. DIY recipes for calming body oils or lotions often include a base of carrier oils paired with essential oils like frankincense or ylang-ylang. These mixtures not only nourish the skin but also allow the calming properties of essential oils to penetrate deeply, providing both physical and emotional benefits. Applying these blends after a bath or before bedtime can further promote a serene state of mind.

Essential oils can also play a role in your cleaning regimen, transforming mundane chores into calming rituals. By incorporating oils such as lemon or eucalyptus into your natural cleaning solutions, you can create a fresh and uplifting atmosphere while keeping your home clean. The aromatic properties of these oils can uplift your mood, making the cleaning process feel less like a chore and more like a self-care activity, thereby enhancing the overall calmness of your living space.

Finally, consider using essential oils in your culinary endeavors to promote relaxation from within. Oils like peppermint or lemon can be added to beverages or dishes, providing not only flavor but also potential wellness benefits. A warm cup of chamomile tea infused with a drop of chamomile essential oil can create a peaceful moment in your day. By consciously incorporating essential oils into various aspects of your life, you can craft an environment that supports relaxation, wellness, and balance, making your space a true sanctuary for both mind and body.

Blends for Focus and Clarity

In the quest for improved focus and mental clarity, essential oils offer a natural and effective solution. Aromatherapy blends can harness the power of specific essential oils known for their cognitive-enhancing properties. Oils such as rosemary, peppermint, and lemon are particularly effective in promoting alertness and concentration. When blended thoughtfully, these oils can create an uplifting and invigorating aroma that not only enhances mood but also aids in mental performance, making them ideal for those engaged in study, work, or creative endeavors.

To craft a blend that enhances focus, consider starting with a base of rosemary essential oil. Renowned for its ability to improve memory retention and stimulate mental activity, rosemary serves as a perfect foundation. Complement this with peppermint essential oil, which is known to invigorate the mind and alleviate feelings of fatigue. A few drops of lemon essential oil can add a refreshing note to the blend while simultaneously uplifting spirits. Together, these oils form a powerful synergy that can clear mental fog and enhance cognitive function.

Incorporating these blends into your daily routine can be achieved in various ways. For instance, using a diffuser allows the aromatic molecules to disperse throughout a room, creating an environment conducive to concentration. Alternatively, a personal aromatherapy inhaler can be prepared for on-the-go support, ensuring that you have access to your focus-enhancing blend during busy days. Additionally, consider adding a few drops of your blend to a carrier oil for a topical application, perfect for pulse points during moments that require heightened clarity.

The application of essential oils for focus and clarity extends beyond mere inhalation. These oils can be incorporated into DIY skincare recipes, creating soothing and aromatic facial mists or creams that not only nurture the skin but also promote alertness throughout the day. By blending essential oils with natural ingredients like aloe vera or witch hazel, you can craft skincare products that serve dual purposes, enhancing both mental sharpness and skin health.

As you explore the realm of essential oils, it's essential to remain mindful of your personal preferences and sensitivities. Conducting patch tests and researching individual oils can help tailor your blends to your specific needs. With the right combinations, essential oils can serve as powerful allies in your pursuit of focus and clarity, enriching your daily life with natural aromas that uplift and inspire.

Rituals Incorporating Essential Oils

Rituals incorporating essential oils can transform everyday activities into meaningful experiences, enhancing both mental and physical well-being. The practice of using essential oils in rituals dates back centuries and has been embraced in various cultures for their therapeutic properties. Integrating essential oils into your daily routine can foster a sense of mindfulness and intentionality, whether you're seeking relaxation, rejuvenation, or a boost to your immune system. By understanding how to blend and utilize these potent natural extracts, you can create personalized rituals that resonate with your individual needs and lifestyle.

One of the simplest ways to incorporate essential oils into your rituals is through aromatherapy. Diffusing essential oils like lavender or eucalyptus can create a calming atmosphere conducive to meditation or relaxation. You might establish a daily practice where you begin or end your day with a few drops of your chosen essential oil in a diffuser, allowing the soothing scents to fill your space. This practice not only promotes a serene environment but also helps to clear your mind and enhance your focus, making it easier to engage in mindfulness or meditation.

For those interested in skincare, creating DIY essential oil blends can elevate your beauty rituals. By combining essential oils such as tea tree, frankincense, or geranium with carrier oils, you can craft personalized serums or moisturizers that address specific skin concerns. Incorporating these blends into your skincare routine can transform a mundane task into a restorative ritual. For example, taking a few moments each evening to apply a nourishing oil blend can serve as a form of self-care, promoting not only healthier skin but also a more relaxed state of mind.

When it comes to cleaning, essential oils can infuse your home with delightful fragrances while providing natural antibacterial properties. Creating a cleaning ritual involving essential oil-infused solutions can make household chores feel more enjoyable and less burdensome. For instance, a blend of lemon and tea tree oil in a spray bottle can not only disinfect surfaces but also uplift your spirit as you clean. This approach allows you to create a healthier environment while promoting a sense of accomplishment and clarity in your living space.

Finally, consider integrating essential oils into your culinary practices as a way to elevate your meals and promote wellness. Using oils like oregano, basil, or peppermint can add depth to your dishes while offering health benefits such as improved digestion or immune support. Developing a ritual around cooking with essential oils encourages creativity in the kitchen and fosters a connection to the food you consume. By being intentional about the ingredients you use and the scents you incorporate, you can create nourishing meals that delight the senses and support your overall well-being.

Chapter 9: Essential Oils for Seasonal Allergies

Understanding Allergies and Their Triggers

Understanding allergies is crucial for anyone interested in incorporating essential oils into their daily routines. Allergies occur when the immune system reacts to substances, known as allergens, that are typically harmless to most people. Common allergens include pollen, dust mites, mold, pet dander, certain foods, and various chemicals. For those utilizing essential oils in their wellness practices, recognizing these triggers is vital to ensure a safe and beneficial experience. Essential oils can provide therapeutic benefits, but they can also exacerbate allergies if one is sensitive to the components within certain oils.

Various essential oils possess properties that may either alleviate or trigger allergic reactions. For example, oils like lavender and eucalyptus are often celebrated for their soothing effects, particularly in helping to relieve symptoms associated with seasonal allergies. However, individuals with sensitivities to these plants may experience irritation or allergic responses. It is essential to understand the specific constituents of each oil, as some compounds can provoke allergies in susceptible individuals. Researching and doing patch tests before full application can help identify potential reactions.

In the realm of DIY skincare recipes, selecting essential oils requires careful consideration. While oils such as tea tree and chamomile are renowned for their skin-soothing properties, they may also cause reactions in individuals prone to allergies. Understanding your skin type and any existing sensitivities is important before incorporating these oils into your regimen. A mindful approach to blending essential oils for skincare can enhance benefits while minimizing the risk of allergic reactions. Always begin with lower concentrations and observe how your skin responds over time.

For those looking to create natural cleaning solutions, it's equally important to be aware of potential allergens. Many essential oils, such as lemon or tea tree, have antibacterial and antifungal properties, making them excellent choices for cleaning. However, some individuals may find themselves sensitive to the strong scents or chemical compositions within these oils. When formulating cleaning solutions, consider using blends that are gentle yet effective, ensuring that the chosen oils do not trigger adverse reactions for household members, including pets.

Incorporating essential oils into culinary recipes, meditation practices, or home fragrance diffusers can also be influenced by a clear understanding of allergies. For culinary uses, oils like peppermint and lemon can add flavor but may not be suitable for everyone. Similarly, during meditation or relaxation practices, oils that promote tranquility should be chosen with care to avoid any unpleasant reactions. Ultimately, being informed about allergies and their triggers allows individuals to not only enjoy the myriad benefits of essential oils but also to do so safely and effectively, enhancing their overall well-being.

Essential Oils to Alleviate Allergy Symptoms

Essential oils have gained popularity as natural remedies for a variety of ailments, including seasonal allergies. Many individuals seeking alternative solutions find that these concentrated plant extracts can provide relief from common allergy symptoms such as nasal congestion, sneezing, and itchy eyes. Certain essential oils possess anti-inflammatory, antihistamine, and soothing properties that can help alleviate discomfort associated with allergic reactions, making them a useful addition to any wellness routine.

Eucalyptus oil is known for its ability to open up the airways and promote easier breathing. Its natural decongestant properties make it particularly effective during allergy season when pollen and other allergens are prevalent. By diffusing eucalyptus oil in your living space or adding a few drops to a warm bath, you can create an environment that supports respiratory health. Additionally, combining eucalyptus with peppermint oil can enhance its effectiveness, as peppermint may help relieve headaches that sometimes accompany allergies.

Lavender oil is another essential oil that can provide significant allergy relief. Its calming scent not only helps to reduce stress, which can exacerbate allergy symptoms, but it also has properties that can alleviate inflammation and irritation in the respiratory system. Incorporating lavender oil into your nighttime routine, whether through a calming diffuser blend or a DIY skincare recipe, can promote relaxation and improve sleep quality, both of which are beneficial for overall immune function during allergy season.

Tea tree oil is revered for its antiseptic and anti-inflammatory properties, making it a valuable ally against allergies. When diluted and applied topically, it can help soothe itchy skin and rashes that may arise from allergic reactions. Additionally, tea tree oil can be added to natural cleaning solutions to help eliminate dust mites and mold, common triggers for allergy sufferers. By creating a cleaner living environment, you can further reduce your exposure to allergens and enhance your overall health.

Lastly, incorporating essential oils like lemon and chamomile into your culinary recipes can also support allergy relief. Lemon oil is rich in antioxidants and can aid in detoxification, while chamomile has a calming effect that can help ease allergy-related anxiety. Both oils can be safely used in food and beverages, providing not just flavor but also additional health benefits. By integrating these essential oils into your daily routine, you can create a comprehensive approach to managing allergy symptoms naturally and effectively.

Blending for Relief

Creating essential oil blends can provide significant relief for various physical and emotional concerns. Understanding the properties of different essential oils allows individuals to craft personalized blends that target specific needs. For those seeking alternative natural products, essential oils can effectively alleviate stress, enhance mood, and promote overall well-being. By exploring the unique characteristics of each oil, one can create combinations that not only smell delightful but also deliver therapeutic benefits.

In the realm of skincare, essential oils can be integrated into DIY recipes to address various skin concerns. Tea tree oil is a potent antiseptic known for its ability to combat acne, while chamomile can soothe irritated skin. Blending these two oils with a carrier oil, such as jojoba or sweet almond oil, creates a nourishing treatment that not only addresses skin issues but also provides a moment of self-care. This approach allows individuals to customize their skincare routine while utilizing the healing properties of nature.

Essential oils also play a vital role in natural cleaning solutions. Oils like lemon and eucalyptus possess antibacterial and antiviral properties, making them ideal for creating effective household cleaners. By blending these oils with vinegar or baking soda, individuals can formulate powerful cleaning agents that are safe for both their homes and the environment. This method not only reduces exposure to harsh chemicals but also infuses the home with refreshing scents that uplift the atmosphere.

For those concerned with wellness and immune support, certain essential oils can play a pivotal role in maintaining health. Oils like oregano and thyme are known for their antimicrobial properties, making them excellent additions to blends aimed at boosting immunity. Incorporating these oils into daily routines, whether through inhalation in a diffuser or diluted in a topical application, can help strengthen the body's defenses. By embracing the art of blending, individuals can create holistic remedies that support their health and enhance their quality of life.

Chapter 10: Essential Oils for Hair Care Treatments

Essential Oils for Different Hair Types

Essential oils have gained popularity for their versatile applications in hair care, offering natural solutions tailored to various hair types. Understanding the unique needs of different hair types is crucial when selecting essential oils, as each type has its distinct characteristics and challenges. This subchapter will explore how essential oils can benefit straight, wavy, curly, and coily hair, providing readers with informed choices for enhancing their hair care routines through natural, aromatic solutions.

For straight hair, essential oils can help maintain shine and manage oil production. Oils such as lavender and rosemary are particularly effective. Lavender oil is known for its calming properties and can promote a healthy scalp, reducing dandruff and excess oil. Rosemary oil enhances circulation, stimulating hair follicles and encouraging growth. A blend of these oils in a carrier oil can be massaged into the scalp for nourishing treatment, leaving straight hair looking vibrant and healthy.

Wavy hair often requires hydration and definition to enhance its natural texture. Essential oils like ylang-ylang and geranium can be beneficial in this regard. Ylang-ylang oil is excellent for balancing moisture levels, preventing frizz while imparting a soft shine. Geranium oil not only helps regulate oil production but also strengthens hair strands, reducing breakage. Incorporating these oils into a leave-in conditioner or hair serum can help define waves and keep them soft and manageable.

Curly hair tends to be more prone to dryness, making it essential to focus on moisturizing and soothing properties. Essential oils such as jojoba and coconut oil are excellent carriers for oils like tea tree and chamomile. Tea tree oil can help maintain a healthy scalp by combating dandruff and irritation, while chamomile oil soothes and hydrates curls. A DIY deep conditioning mask using these oils can provide the moisture and nourishment that curly hair craves, promoting bounce and vitality.

Coily hair requires the most moisture and protection due to its structure, which makes it prone to dryness and breakage. Essential oils such as peppermint and cedarwood are ideal for stimulating hair growth and providing a soothing effect on the scalp. Peppermint oil creates a refreshing sensation that can help increase blood flow to the scalp, while cedarwood oil strengthens hair and provides a grounding aroma. Blending these oils into a rich, heavy conditioner can create a luxurious treatment that enhances the health and appearance of coily hair.

In summary, selecting the right essential oils for different hair types can significantly enhance hair health and appearance. By understanding the needs of straight, wavy, curly, and coily hair, individuals can create personalized blends that not only address specific challenges but also provide therapeutic benefits. Incorporating essential oils into hair care routines allows for a holistic approach, aligning with the principles of natural products and their effectiveness in promoting overall wellness.

Homemade Hair Treatments and Masks

Homemade hair treatments and masks offer a fantastic way to nourish and revitalize your hair using natural ingredients, particularly when combined with the powerful properties of essential oils. These treatments can address various hair concerns, such as dryness, frizz, and lack of shine, while also promoting a healthy scalp. The beauty of DIY hair care lies in its customization; you can tailor the ingredients to suit your specific needs, making it an ideal choice for those seeking alternative natural products.

Coconut oil is a popular base for many hair masks due to its moisturizing properties and ability to penetrate the hair shaft. When combined with essential oils like lavender or rosemary, this blend not only hydrates but also enhances scalp health and stimulates hair growth. For an added boost, consider mixing a few drops of tea tree oil, known for its antifungal and antibacterial properties, which can help alleviate dandruff and maintain a clean scalp. This simple yet effective mask can be applied once a week for optimal results.

For those with oily hair or scalp, a treatment featuring apple cider vinegar and essential oils can provide a refreshing and balancing effect. Apple cider vinegar helps to remove buildup while restoring pH balance. Adding essential oils such as peppermint or lemon can invigorate the scalp and leave your hair feeling fresh and clean. This combination not only helps to clarify but also adds a delightful aroma, making your hair care routine a truly aromatic experience.

Deep conditioning is essential for maintaining healthy hair, especially for those with color-treated or heat-damaged strands. A nourishing mask made from avocado and honey can work wonders. Avocado is rich in vitamins and fatty acids, while honey acts as a natural humectant that locks in moisture. Incorporating essential oils such as ylang-ylang or geranium can provide additional hydration and enhance shine. This luxurious treatment can be left on for 20-30 minutes before rinsing, allowing your hair to absorb all the nourishing benefits.

Finally, incorporating essential oils into your hair treatments can also enhance your overall wellness. Using calming oils like chamomile or sandalwood in your mask can create a soothing experience that not only benefits your hair but also promotes relaxation. This dual approach of nurturing your hair while indulging in aromatherapy can transform your self-care routine into a holistic practice, making homemade hair treatments not just a beauty regimen but a moment of tranquility as well.

Recipes for Scalp Health

The health of your scalp plays a crucial role in the overall condition of your hair, and incorporating essential oils into your hair care routine can provide a natural solution to maintain scalp health. There are a variety of essential oils known for their beneficial properties that can help alleviate issues such as dryness, itchiness, and dandruff. In this section, we will explore several effective recipes that utilize these oils to promote a healthy scalp, focusing on natural ingredients that are easily accessible and simple to use.

One of the most popular essential oils for scalp health is tea tree oil. Renowned for its antifungal and antibacterial properties, tea tree oil can help combat dandruff and soothe irritation. To create a scalp treatment, mix five drops of tea tree oil with two tablespoons of a carrier oil like jojoba or coconut oil. Apply this blend directly to your scalp, massaging it in gently. Leave it on for at least 30 minutes before rinsing with a mild shampoo. This treatment can be done once a week to maintain a balanced and healthy scalp environment.

Another excellent choice is lavender essential oil, which is celebrated for its calming effects and ability to promote hair growth. To create a calming scalp infusion, combine three drops of lavender oil with two tablespoons of sweet almond oil. Massage the mixture into your scalp and allow it to sit for about an hour. This recipe not only nourishes the scalp but also provides a relaxing aromatherapy experience. Incorporating this treatment into your routine can help alleviate stress while promoting a healthy hair growth cycle.

For those dealing with oily scalps, rosemary essential oil can be particularly beneficial. Known for its stimulating properties, rosemary oil can enhance circulation to the scalp and help regulate oil production. To make a balancing scalp treatment, blend four drops of rosemary oil with two tablespoons of apple cider vinegar and two tablespoons of water. Apply this mixture to your scalp after shampooing, leaving it on for a few minutes before rinsing thoroughly. This natural rinse helps maintain a clean and healthy scalp, providing a refreshing alternative to commercial products.

Finally, incorporating essential oils into your regular conditioning routine can further enhance scalp health. A nourishing scalp mask can be created by mixing three drops of peppermint oil with half a ripe avocado and two tablespoons of honey. Blend the ingredients until smooth and apply the mask directly to your scalp and hair. Leave it on for 20 minutes before washing it out with a gentle shampoo. This recipe not only hydrates the scalp but also invigorates the senses, making it a delightful addition to your hair care regimen. By using these natural recipes, you can embrace the power of essential oils for a healthier scalp and more vibrant hair.

Chapter 11: Essential Oils for Home Fragrance Diffusers

Choosing the Right Essential Oils for Your Space

Choosing the right essential oils for your space involves understanding the unique benefits and properties of various oils, as well as how they can enhance your environment. Essential oils can serve multiple purposes, from promoting relaxation and wellness to providing natural cleaning solutions and uplifting home fragrances. When selecting oils, consider your specific needs and the atmosphere you wish to create. This foundational knowledge will help you make informed decisions that align with your lifestyle.

For aromatherapy blends, focus on oils known for their therapeutic effects. Lavender is often favored for its calming properties, making it ideal for relaxation and stress relief. In contrast, citrus oils like lemon and orange are energizing and can uplift your mood. If you seek to enhance your meditation practice, consider using frankincense or sandalwood, which promote a sense of tranquility and grounding. Understanding the emotional and physical responses elicited by different oils can significantly enhance your experience.

When creating DIY essential oil skincare recipes, it is crucial to choose oils that not only smell pleasant but also offer skin benefits. Tea tree oil is renowned for its antibacterial properties, making it suitable for acne treatment, while rose oil is celebrated for its hydrating qualities. For a soothing blend, consider chamomile or lavender oil, which can help calm irritated skin. Ensuring that the oils you choose are compatible with your skin type will enhance the effectiveness of your skincare regimen.

For those interested in natural cleaning solutions, essential oils can serve as powerful agents. Oils like tea tree, eucalyptus, and lemon possess antimicrobial properties, making them excellent choices for disinfecting surfaces. Additionally, adding a few drops of these oils to your cleaning routine can leave a refreshing aroma, transforming mundane chores into a more enjoyable experience. When selecting oils for cleaning, consider their scent and effectiveness to create a cleaner that not only works well but also makes your home smell inviting.

Incorporating essential oils into your daily life can also extend to culinary uses, pet care, and hair treatments. Oils such as peppermint and basil can enhance flavor in dishes, while oils like chamomile can promote relaxation when used in teas. In pet care, always ensure that the oils you choose are safe for animals, as some can be harmful. For hair treatments, oils like rosemary and lavender can stimulate growth and improve scalp health. By thoughtfully selecting essential oils for various applications, you can create a harmonious and holistic environment that supports your overall well-being.

Blending Techniques for Diffusers

Blending techniques for diffusers play a crucial role in maximizing the benefits of essential oils. As individuals seek alternative natural products for various applications, understanding the art of blending can significantly enhance the experience of using essential oils for aromatherapy. A well-crafted blend not only delivers an appealing fragrance but also supports emotional and physical wellness. By experimenting with various combinations, you can create unique fragrances that resonate with your personal preferences and desired outcomes.

When creating diffuser blends, it is essential to consider the top, middle, and base notes of essential oils. Top notes are the first scents you smell, often bright and uplifting, like citrus oils. Middle notes provide balance and depth, with floral or herbal characteristics. Base notes are grounding and long-lasting, such as woods or resins. A harmonious blend usually contains a mix of these notes, creating a more complex and satisfying aroma. For instance, combining lemon (top), lavender (middle), and cedarwood (base) can yield a refreshing yet calming experience, ideal for meditation and relaxation.

In addition to the aromatic profile, the therapeutic properties of each essential oil should guide your blending process. For those focused on wellness and immune support, oils like eucalyptus, tea tree, and oregano can be combined for their antibacterial and antiviral properties. Conversely, if you are targeting seasonal allergies, consider blending peppermint, lavender, and lemon to create a refreshing and soothing atmosphere. Understanding the unique benefits of each oil allows you to tailor your blends to address specific needs effectively.

Another significant factor in blending techniques is the method of diffusion. Different diffusers, whether ultrasonic, nebulizing, or heat-based, can influence how the oils disperse into the air. Ultrasonic diffusers, for example, work well with blends that have a higher water content, while nebulizing diffusers are ideal for potent, undiluted oils. When crafting your blends, consider how the method of diffusion may alter the aroma and therapeutic effects. This knowledge enables you to create recipes that are not only pleasant but also effective for your intended purpose, such as natural cleaning solutions or pet care.

Lastly, keep in mind the importance of personal experimentation in the blending process. Each individual's preference for scents and their experiences with essential oils can vary widely. Start with basic blends that appeal to your senses, then gradually modify the proportions or introduce new oils. Document your creations, noting which combinations work best for you in different contexts, such as cooking or skincare. This practice not only enhances your understanding of essential oils but also empowers you to develop personalized blends that cater to your unique lifestyle, ultimately enriching your journey with natural products.

Seasonal Fragrance Recipes

Seasonal fragrances can significantly enhance our mood and environment, making them an essential component of our aromatic repertoire. As the seasons change, so too does our need for different scents that resonate with the atmosphere around us. Essential oils offer a versatile way to create blends that not only smell delightful but also provide various physical and emotional benefits. This subchapter will explore a selection of seasonal fragrance recipes tailored to enhance well-being, invigorate our spaces, and harmonize with the rhythms of nature.

In spring, we often seek scents that embody renewal and freshness. A blend of lemon, lavender, and eucalyptus can create a vibrant atmosphere that mirrors the blossoming flowers and budding greenery. Lemon's uplifting aroma is invigorating, while lavender promotes relaxation and balance. Eucalyptus adds a crisp, refreshing note that can help clear the mind and support respiratory health, making this blend ideal for diffusing during spring cleaning or when welcoming guests. Additionally, this combination serves as a wonderful base for DIY skincare recipes, providing a refreshing toner that can invigorate the complexion.

As summer approaches, the desire for light, fruity, and floral fragrances becomes more prominent. A blend of sweet orange, ylang-ylang, and geranium captures the essence of sunny days and blooming gardens. Sweet orange is known for its cheerful and uplifting properties, while ylang-ylang adds a touch of exotic sweetness that can help reduce stress and anxiety. Geranium provides a balancing effect, promoting emotional stability. This blend is not only perfect for home fragrance diffusers but can also be incorporated into natural cleaning solutions, ensuring your home smells fresh and inviting during summer gatherings.

With the arrival of autumn, the air becomes crisp, and the leaves turn vibrant hues, prompting a shift in our fragrance preferences. A warming blend of cedarwood, cinnamon, and clove creates a cozy atmosphere reminiscent of fall festivities. Cedarwood offers grounding properties, while cinnamon and clove bring warmth and spice, supporting feelings of comfort and security. This blend can be particularly effective in promoting relaxation during meditation and can be used in hair care treatments to impart a warm, inviting scent while nourishing the scalp. Additionally, it serves as a natural remedy for seasonal allergies, soothing the respiratory system.

Winter often calls for deeper, richer scents that evoke the spirit of the season. A combination of frankincense, pine, and bergamot can transform your environment into a tranquil winter retreat. Frankincense is renowned for its grounding and meditative qualities, making it perfect for times of reflection. Pine evokes the fresh scent of evergreen trees and can help boost immunity during the colder months. Bergamot adds a bright note that lifts the spirits and combats winter blues. This blend works beautifully in diffusers or can be incorporated into wellness rituals, creating a calming atmosphere perfect for relaxation and self-care.

These seasonal fragrance recipes illustrate the power of essential oils to enhance our lives in various ways. By selecting the right blends for each season, we can not only enjoy the aromatic benefits but also tap into the therapeutic properties that essential oils offer. Whether you are looking to create an inviting atmosphere in your home, support your wellness journey, or simply enjoy the seasonal changes through scent, these recipes provide an excellent starting point for your aromatic alchemy.

Chapter 12: Conclusion and Next Steps

Embracing Aromatic Alchemy in Daily Life

Embracing aromatic alchemy in daily life involves integrating essential oils into various aspects of your routine, enhancing both your physical and emotional well-being. Essential oils are versatile and can be used for a myriad of purposes, from aromatherapy to skincare, and even culinary applications. By understanding the unique properties of different oils, you can create personalized blends that cater to your specific needs, making aromatic alchemy an enriching practice that transforms everyday experiences.

Incorporating essential oils into your skincare regimen can be both simple and rewarding. DIY essential oil skincare recipes allow you to craft natural products that are free from synthetic ingredients. For instance, combining lavender oil with a carrier oil provides a soothing moisturizer, while tea tree oil can be added to treat blemishes. Exploring the world of essential oils enables you to tailor your skincare routine, addressing concerns such as dryness, oiliness, or acne, all while nourishing your skin naturally.

Essential oils also play a significant role in creating a cleaner, healthier home environment. By utilizing oils such as lemon, eucalyptus, or tea tree in DIY natural cleaning solutions, you can effectively eliminate germs and odors without resorting to harsh chemicals. These natural alternatives not only promote a clean living space but also infuse your home with delightful aromas, contributing to a refreshing atmosphere. Embracing this approach not only prioritizes your health but also supports a more sustainable lifestyle.

For those interested in wellness and immune support, essential oils like oregano, eucalyptus, and peppermint can be beneficial. Incorporating these oils into your daily routine, whether through diffusion, topical application, or even culinary recipes, can help bolster your immune system and enhance your overall vitality. Additionally, these oils can be particularly effective in alleviating symptoms related to seasonal allergies, providing relief through their natural antihistamine properties.

Lastly, the use of essential oils extends to mental and emotional wellness, particularly in practices like meditation and relaxation. Oils such as frankincense and chamomile can create a serene environment, promoting tranquility and focus. Incorporating these oils into your meditation practice can enhance the experience, allowing you to delve deeper into mindfulness. Furthermore, essential oils can be used in home fragrance diffusers to create an inviting and calming atmosphere, making your living space a sanctuary of peace and comfort. Embracing aromatic alchemy in daily life not only enriches your routines but also fosters a deeper connection to nature and well-being.

Resources for Further Exploration

For those interested in diving deeper into the world of essential oils and their myriad applications, a wealth of resources is available to guide and enhance your journey. Numerous books dedicated to essential oils and aromatherapy can provide in-depth knowledge and practical advice. Titles such as "The Complete Book of Essential Oils and Aromatherapy" by Valerie Ann Worwood offer a comprehensive overview, including detailed descriptions of specific oils, their properties, and suggested uses. Additionally, "Essential Oil Safety" by Robert Tisserand and Rodney Young presents crucial safety information, ensuring that users understand proper dilution rates and contraindications, particularly important for those exploring DIY skincare and household cleaning solutions.

Online platforms serve as another invaluable resource for enthusiasts seeking alternative natural products. Websites such as the National Association for Holistic Aromatherapy (NAHA) provide a plethora of articles, research papers, and guidelines on essential oil usage. These resources cover a wide range of topics, from the best practices for creating effective aromatherapy blends to detailed instructions for incorporating essential oils into culinary recipes. Many reputable essential oil suppliers also maintain blogs filled with creative ideas, tips, and recipes that cater to various needs, such as wellness support, pet care, and seasonal allergy relief.

Community forums and social media groups dedicated to essential oils can also facilitate knowledge sharing and personal experiences among users. Engaging with like-minded individuals allows you to gain insights into practical applications and receive recommendations for products and methods that work best. Platforms such as Facebook and Instagram often feature influencers and educators who share their expertise in essential oils, offering tutorials, videos, and live sessions that enhance understanding and inspire creativity. These interactive spaces can be particularly beneficial for those exploring essential oils for meditation, relaxation, and home fragrance diffusers.

For those who prefer hands-on learning, workshops and classes provide an excellent opportunity to experiment with essential oils under the guidance of experienced practitioners. Many local health stores, wellness centers, and essential oil distributors offer workshops that cover topics ranging from basic blending techniques to advanced applications in skincare or natural cleaning. Participating in these sessions can enhance your practical skills, allowing you to confidently create personalized blends tailored to your specific needs, whether they be for hair care treatments or immune support.

Lastly, podcasts and YouTube channels dedicated to essential oils can be an engaging way to absorb information while multitasking. Many experts in the field share their insights, tips, and experiences through these mediums, making it easy to learn about new applications or trends in essential oil usage. Listening to interviews with aromatherapy professionals or watching demonstrations of DIY recipes can serve as a source of inspiration and motivation, encouraging you to experiment with essential oils in various aspects of your life, from culinary endeavors to natural wellness practices.

Final Thoughts on Natural Living

Natural living is a holistic approach that encourages individuals to embrace a lifestyle centered around natural products and practices. By integrating essential oils into daily routines, one can enhance not only personal well-being but also the environment. Essential oils, derived from plants, offer a multitude of benefits that align with the principles of natural living. They can be used in various applications, from skincare to home cleaning, promoting health and sustainability in everyday life.

When exploring essential oils for aromatherapy blends, it's important to understand how different oils can impact mood and emotional well-being. Oils like lavender and chamomile are renowned for their calming properties, making them ideal for relaxation and stress relief. In contrast, invigorating oils such as lemon and peppermint can uplift the spirit and enhance focus. Crafting personalized blends allows individuals to harness the therapeutic potential of these oils, creating an aromatic experience tailored to their specific needs.

DIY essential oil skincare recipes represent another facet of natural living that empowers individuals to take control of their health. By using essential oils in homemade skincare products, one can avoid the chemicals and preservatives often found in commercial products. Ingredients like tea tree oil can combat blemishes, while rosehip oil provides essential nutrients for the skin. These natural alternatives not only promote healthier skin but also align with the ethos of sustainability by reducing reliance on mass-produced goods.

Incorporating essential oils into cleaning solutions is a practical way to enhance home environments while minimizing exposure to harsh chemicals. Oils like tea tree and eucalyptus possess natural antibacterial properties, making them effective for disinfecting surfaces. By creating DIY cleaning products, individuals can maintain a clean home while supporting their commitment to natural living. This approach not only improves indoor air quality but also fosters a sense of well-being for all inhabitants.

Finally, the versatility of essential oils extends to culinary uses, pet care, and wellness support, making them indispensable in a natural living lifestyle. From flavoring dishes to enhancing meditation practices, essential oils can elevate experiences and promote overall health. Their ability to support immune function and alleviate seasonal allergies further exemplifies their role in fostering wellness. Embracing essential oils in these various applications not only enriches individual lives but also encourages a more sustainable and health-conscious approach to living.